Table of Contents

Introduction

After experiencing a stroke, proper nutrition is critical to aid in the recovery process. The right foods can help with brain function, energy levels, and overall well-being. This is why The Stroke Recovery Cookbook was created - to provide delicious and nutritious recipes that can assist in regaining health and wellness after a stroke.

This chapter will explore the role of food in stroke recovery and provide an overview of the important nutrients that are needed during this time. It will also discuss the challenges that stroke survivors may face when it comes to eating and offer tips for making mealtime easier and more enjoyable.

The Importance of Nutrition in Stroke Recovery

Stroke recovery can be a long and challenging process, and nutrition plays a crucial role in the healing journey. Eating a balanced diet that is rich in vitamins, minerals, and antioxidants can help to reduce inflammation, support brain function, and aid in the repair of damaged tissues. Good nutrition can also help to manage other health conditions that may be related to stroke, such as high blood pressure, diabetes, and high cholesterol.

Important Nutrients for Stroke Recovery

There are several key nutrients that are particularly important for stroke recovery, including:

1. Omega-3 Fatty Acids - These healthy fats are found in fish, nuts, and seeds and have been shown to have anti-inflammatory properties that can aid in brain function and reduce the risk of stroke.
2. B Vitamins - These vitamins, including B12 and folate, play a crucial role in brain function and can help to reduce the risk of stroke.
3. Vitamin D - This vitamin is essential for bone health and can also aid in brain function and mood regulation.

4. Antioxidants - These substances, found in fruits, vegetables, and whole grains, can help to reduce inflammation and protect against oxidative stress, which can contribute to stroke risk.

Challenges with Eating After a Stroke

Many stroke survivors may experience challenges with eating, such as difficulty swallowing or chewing, changes in taste or smell, and reduced appetite. These challenges can make it difficult to consume the nutrients needed for recovery. In addition, stroke survivors may also have dietary restrictions due to other health conditions, such as high blood pressure or diabetes.

Tips for Eating After a Stroke

Despite the challenges that stroke survivors may face when it comes to eating, there are several tips that can help to make mealtime easier and more enjoyable. These include:

Choose Soft and Easy-to-Swallow Foods - Foods that are soft and easy to swallow, such as pureed soups or mashed potatoes, can be easier for stroke survivors to eat.

Use Seasonings and Herbs - Changes in taste or smell can make food less appealing, but using seasonings and herbs can add flavor and make meals more enjoyable.

Eat Small, Frequent Meals - Eating smaller, more frequent meals throughout the day can make it easier to consume the necessary nutrients without feeling overwhelmed.

Stay Hydrated - Dehydration can exacerbate many stroke-related symptoms, so it is important to drink plenty of fluids throughout the day.

Easy and Nutritious Breakfasts: Starting the Day Right

Breakfast is an important meal of the day, particularly for individuals recovering from stroke. A balanced breakfast provides the necessary energy and nutrients needed to start the day, helps to stabilize blood sugar levels, and supports the brain and body's recovery process. In this chapter, we will explore a variety of easy and nutritious breakfast ideas that are designed to promote optimal healing and wellness.

Oatmeal with Berries and Nuts: Oatmeal is a fantastic source of fiber, which supports digestive health and helps to regulate blood sugar levels. Adding fresh berries and nuts to your oatmeal boosts its nutritional value, providing a range of essential vitamins, minerals, and antioxidants that support brain and body health.

Veggie Omelet: Omelets are an easy and delicious way to pack in a range of nutrients in one meal. Using egg whites or a mixture of whole eggs and egg whites helps to reduce cholesterol intake while still providing essential protein. Adding a variety of vegetables, such as spinach, bell peppers, onions, and mushrooms, provides fiber, vitamins, and minerals that promote optimal brain and body function.

Whole Grain Toast with Peanut Butter and Banana: Whole grain toast provides slow-release carbohydrates that provide sustained energy throughout the morning, while peanut butter provides healthy fats and protein that promote satiety and support brain and body function. Adding sliced banana to your toast provides additional fiber, vitamins, and minerals that support optimal health and wellness.

Greek Yogurt Parfait: Greek yogurt is a fantastic source of protein, calcium, and probiotics, which support optimal brain and body function. Layering it with fresh fruit and granola provides additional fiber, vitamins, and minerals that support optimal digestive health and overall wellness.

Smoothie Bowl: Smoothie bowls are a fun and easy way to pack in a range of essential nutrients in one meal. Combining frozen fruit, vegetables, protein powder, and nut milk in a blender creates a nutrient-dense meal that supports optimal brain and body function. Topping it with fresh fruit, nuts, and seeds provides additional fiber, vitamins, and minerals that support digestive health and overall wellness.

Nourishing Soups and Stews: Comforting and Healing Meals

After a stroke, the body needs nourishing foods that provide essential nutrients to help with recovery. One great way to do this is by enjoying a hot and comforting bowl of soup or stew. These dishes are easy to digest and can be packed with vitamins, minerals, and other nutrients that are essential for healing.

In this chapter, we will explore a variety of soup and stew recipes that are both delicious and nutritious. From classic chicken noodle soup to hearty beef stew, these meals are perfect for those who want to eat well while still enjoying comforting and satisfying food.

Classic Chicken Noodle Soup

This recipe is a classic for a reason. It's easy to make and packed with nutrients that are essential for healing. Chicken is a great source of protein, which is important for repairing and rebuilding muscles. Carrots, celery, and onions provide vitamins and minerals, while egg noodles offer a comforting and satisfying texture. This soup is perfect for those who want a comforting and nourishing meal.

Vegetable Soup

Vegetable soup is a great way to pack in nutrients without adding a lot of calories. This recipe is filled with a variety of vegetables, including carrots, celery, onions, and spinach. These ingredients are loaded with vitamins, minerals, and other nutrients that are important for recovery. Additionally, the broth is made with low-sodium chicken stock, making it a heart-healthy option.

Lentil Soup

Lentils are a great source of protein and fiber, making them an ideal food for those recovering from a stroke. This lentil soup recipe is easy to make and packed with essential nutrients. The lentils are cooked with onions, garlic, carrots, celery, and tomatoes, making it a flavorful and satisfying meal.

Beef Stew

Beef stew is a hearty and satisfying meal that is perfect for those who want a comforting meal. This recipe is packed with vegetables, including carrots, onions, and celery, making it a great source of essential nutrients. Additionally, the beef is slow-cooked, making it tender and easy to digest.

Butternut Squash Soup

Butternut squash is a great source of vitamins A and C, making it an ideal food for those recovering from a stroke. This soup recipe is easy to make and perfect for those who want a comforting and nourishing meal. The butternut squash is cooked with onions, garlic, and chicken stock, creating a flavorful and comforting soup.

Power-Packed Salads: Boosting Energy and Vitality

Salads are a great way to incorporate fresh, nutrient-dense ingredients into your diet. They are packed with fiber, vitamins, and minerals that are essential for maintaining good health. This chapter focuses on creating salads that are not only delicious but also provide the necessary nutrients for stroke recovery.

Understanding the Importance of Salads for Stroke Recovery

Salads are an important part of stroke recovery nutrition as they provide the necessary nutrients for the body to heal and repair. They are a great source of antioxidants, which can help reduce inflammation and oxidative stress in the body. Salads also provide fiber, which can help regulate blood sugar levels and promote healthy digestion. In addition, leafy greens like kale, spinach, and arugula are rich in vitamin K, which is essential for maintaining healthy bones and preventing fractures.

Tips for Creating Power-Packed Salads

Creating a salad that is both delicious and nutritious can be easy if you follow a few simple tips:

Start with a variety of greens: Mix and match different types of greens to create a flavorful and nutrient-dense base for your salad. Some great options include kale, spinach, arugula, romaine, and mixed greens.

Add color with fruits and vegetables: Adding colorful fruits and vegetables not only makes your salad visually appealing but also provides a variety of vitamins and minerals. Some great options include tomatoes, bell peppers, carrots, cucumbers, strawberries, and blueberries.

Incorporate healthy fats: Healthy fats like avocado, nuts, and seeds not only add flavor and texture to your salad but also provide essential nutrients like omega-3 fatty acids and vitamin E.

Choose lean proteins: Adding lean proteins like grilled chicken, tofu, or beans to your salad can help keep you feeling full and satisfied while providing important nutrients for recovery.

Delicious and Nutritious Salad Recipes

This section includes several delicious and nutritious salad recipes that are perfect for stroke recovery. Each recipe includes a list of ingredients and step-by-step instructions for preparation. Some of the recipes include:

Superfood Salad with Grilled Chicken: This salad is packed with superfoods like kale, quinoa, and blueberries, and topped with grilled chicken for a lean protein source.

Mediterranean Chickpea Salad: This salad features chickpeas, cucumber, tomato, and feta cheese, all drizzled with a lemon vinaigrette for a refreshing and flavorful dish.

Asian-Inspired Tofu Salad: This salad features marinated tofu, crunchy veggies, and a homemade sesame dressing for an Asian-inspired flavor.

Spinach and Strawberry Salad with Toasted Almonds: This sweet and savory salad features fresh spinach, sweet strawberries, and crunchy toasted almonds for a delicious and nutrient-packed meal.

By incorporating these salads into your diet, you can provide your body with the necessary nutrients for stroke recovery while also enjoying delicious and satisfying meals

Meal Planning and Prep: Practical Tips for Simplifying Your Recovery Diet

Recovering from a stroke can be a challenging journey, and managing your diet during this time is critical to your overall recovery. Meal planning and preparation can seem daunting, especially if you are already dealing with the physical and emotional demands of stroke recovery. However, with some planning and preparation, you can simplify your recovery diet and make the process easier for yourself.

Assess Your Nutritional Needs

Before you start meal planning and preparation, it is important to assess your nutritional needs. Stroke recovery can involve a variety of physical and cognitive challenges, which can impact your dietary needs. For example, if you have difficulty chewing or swallowing, you may need to modify your diet to include soft foods or pureed meals. Additionally, stroke survivors may experience changes in appetite or difficulty with meal preparation, which can impact their overall nutritional status.

Working with a registered dietitian can help you assess your individual nutritional needs and develop a meal plan that meets your specific requirements. A dietitian can also provide guidance on how to modify recipes to meet your nutritional needs and offer tips for meal preparation.

Create a Meal Plan

Once you have assessed your nutritional needs, the next step is to create a meal plan. Meal planning involves deciding what you will eat for each meal and snack throughout the week. A well-planned meal plan can help ensure that you are meeting your nutritional needs and can save time and money by reducing the need for frequent trips to the grocery store.

When creating a meal plan, consider your dietary requirements, preferences, and lifestyle. For example, if you have a busy schedule, you may want to plan for meals that can be prepared in advance or in bulk.

To simplify your meal planning process, consider using a meal planning app or website, which can generate customized meal plans based on your dietary requirements and preferences.

Prep Your Meals in Advance

Meal preparation involves preparing your meals in advance to make mealtime easier and more convenient. Meal preparation can involve a variety of techniques, such as batch cooking, pre-chopping vegetables, and pre-portioning snacks.

Prepping your meals in advance can help you save time and reduce stress during mealtime. It can also help ensure that you are eating healthy and nutritious meals, even when you are short on time.

To simplify your meal prep process, consider investing in meal prep containers, which can help you portion and store your meals. You can also make use of slow cookers, which allow you to cook large batches of meals with minimal effort.

Incorporate Convenience Foods

While fresh and whole foods are always the best choice, convenience foods can be a helpful addition to your stroke recovery diet. Convenience foods can include frozen vegetables, canned fruits, and pre-cooked meats. These foods can be a helpful addition to your meal plan when you are short on time or energy.

When choosing convenience foods, be sure to read the labels carefully and choose options that are low in sodium and free from added sugars. Additionally, be mindful of portion sizes, as some convenience foods can be high in calories.

Stay Hydrated

Proper hydration is critical for stroke recovery, as it can help reduce the risk of complications such as urinary tract infections and constipation. Additionally, dehydration can impact cognitive function and overall energy levels.

To ensure that you are staying hydrated, aim to drink at least eight glasses of water per day. You can also incorporate other hydrating beverages such as herbal tea and low-sugar fruit juices.

Recipes for stroke recovery 1

Cauliflower Tacos

Ingredients

1 small Head Cauliflower ((about 1 ½ cups))

4 oz Fresh Mushrooms

½ cup Walnuts (use less or omit if watching fat intake)

2 Tbs Soy Sauce

2 Tbs Chili Powder

2 tsp Ground Cumin

1 tsp Smoked Paprika

½ tsp Garlic Powder

½ tsp Onion Powder

¼ tsp Ground Pepper

¼ tsp Salt

Instructions

1. Preheat oven to 350 degrees F

2. Lightly pulse the mushrooms in a food processor until you have a rice like consistency

3. Now pulse (or chop) the walnuts to the same consistency and mix in a large bowl

4. Remove the core and leaves of your cauliflower and cut into small pieces

5. Pulse the cauliflower to the same consistency and add to bowl

6. Stir in soy sauce and mix

7. Stir in spices and mix well, making sure everything is mixed thoroughly

8. Spread mixture onto a parchment lined baking sheet and bake for 30 minutes

9. Stir lightly and continue baking for an additional 10-15 minutes

Hot and Sour Soup

Ingredients

2 cups Low Sodium Vegetable Broth

1 cup Water

8 oz Tofu ((extra firm))

8 oz Shiitake Mushrooms

4 oz Bamboo Shoots ((optional))

3 Tbs Low Sodium Soy Sauce

3 Tbs Rice Vinegar

1 Tbs Hoisin Sauce

½ tsp Huy Fong Chili Garlic Sauce ((or more to taste))

⅛ tsp White Pepper

3 Tbs Cornstarch

3 Tbs Water

Instructions

1. Drain Tofu and wrap in towels. Cover with something heavy and allow to press for 5-10 minutes. Then cut into ¾" cubes.

2. Rinse and de-stem mushrooms, then slice into strips. Set aside.

3. Bring 2 cups of Low Sodium Vegetable Broth and 1 cup of Water to a slow boil in a large soup pot.

4. Add mushrooms, tofu, bamboo shoots, soy sauce, and hoisin. Stir to combine. Let simmer for 3-5 minutes.

5. Stir in vinegar, chili sauce, and pepper. Continue simmering for 1-2 minutes.

6. Whisk cornstarch and water together to make a slurry then stir into soup. It should begin to thicken immediately.

7. Stir well and simmer until thickened.

Stir Fry Ever

Ingredients

The Sauce

¼ cup low-sodium vegetable broth

¼ cup low-sodium soy sauce (or tamari)

2 Tbs rice vinegar

2 Tbs maple syrup

1 Tbs minced garlic

1 Tbs minced ginger

3 tsp sriracha

1 Tbs corn starch

The Stir Fry

1 cup of sauce

12-14 oz package extra firm organic tofu (optional)

1 lb baby bella mushrooms (optional)

12 oz package frozen stir fry vegetables

Instructions

1. Add all the sauce ingredients to a mason jar, attach lid, and shake thoroughly

2. If using tofu in your stir fry, press first to remove as much moisture as possible, then cut into cubes

3. Use a 1 qt mason jar to marinate tofu cubes with the sauce - at least 1 hour

4. Drain tofu and reserve sauce.

5. Bake or air fry the tofu - 375°F - about 20 minutes total - flipping midway

6. Clean mushrooms and cut in half

7. Add mushrooms to wok with a splash of veg broth or water - turn heat to high

8. Once broth begins to boil, add frozen veggies and stir-fry juat a few minutes - until crisp-tender

9. Add baked tofu cubes and remaining sauce

10. Stir until sauce has thickened

11. Serve over your favorite rice

Red Chile Sauce

Ingredients

20 New Mexico Red Chile Pods ((dried))

¼ tsp Salt

½ tsp Cumin

½ tsp Mexican Oregano

½ tsp Onion Powder

½ tsp Garlic Powder

2-3 cloves Garlic

1 can Tomato Sauce ((8oz))

2 cups Water

2 cups Water

Instructions

1. Preheat oven to 250 degrees F.

2. Arrange 20 chile pods on a cookie sheet and roast for 20 minutes

3. Flip chiles halfway through roasting process

4. After chiles have cooled to touch,remove stems and seeds

5. Add chiles and onion to large pasta pot and cover with water

6. Bring to a boil, then reduce heat, cover, and simmer for 10 minutes

7. Strain the chiles if desired, or reserve 2 cups of water for blending

8. Carefully remove chiles and onion from pot and add to blender

9. Add remaining ingredients and blend until smooth

Whole Wheat Chocolate Zucchini Bread

INGREDIENTS

1 cup Whole Wheat Flour

½ cup Cocoa Powder

½ teaspoon Baking powder

¾ teaspoon Baking soda

¼ teaspoon Salt

1 cup Zucchini grated, packed

⅓ cup Avocado oil

¼ cup Greek Yogurt

½ cup Sugar granulated

2 Eggs large, room temperature

1 teaspoon Vanilla extract

¾ cup Chocolate chips

Instructions

1. Pre-heat the oven at 350°F. Grease a 4x8 inch loaf pan or line a parchment paper in the pan.

2. Take a large bowl and add the dry ingredients – whole wheat flour, cocoa powder, baking soda, baking powder and salt. Once you have mixed all the dry ingredients well, set them aside.

3. Take another large bowl and add the grated zucchini along with yogurt, oil, sugar, eggs, and vanilla extract. Mix all of them together.

4. Then fold the dry ingredients in to the wet ingredients with a spatula. Do not overmix.

5. At last, add those chocolate chips for that chocolaty goodness. Save some of the chocolate chips to add on top of the batter once you have poured it into the pan.

6. Pour the batter into the prepared baking pan. Spread the chocolate chips evenly over the batter.

7. Slide the pan into the oven and bake for up to 40-50 minutes or until done. Insert a toothpick to check whether the bread is done. If the toothpick comes out clean, take out the pan and let it cool for about 10 minutes.

8. Remove the zucchini bread from the pan and place it on the wire rack.

9. Slice and enjoy this healthy zucchini bread.

Spaghetti with Balsamic Roasted Tomatoes

INGREDIENTS

5 cups (1.25 L) halved cherry tomatoes

2 cups (500 mL) cooked chickpeas (if using canned, be sure to thoroughly rinse)

4 garlic cloves, smashed

3 tbsp (45 mL) canola oil

3 tbsp (45 mL) balsamic vinegar

1/4 tsp (1 mL) black pepper

1 box (13 oz/375 g) whole grain spaghetti

1/2 cup (125 mL) chopped fresh basil, plus more for garnish

Optional garnish: 1/4 cup (60 mL) crumbled feta cheese or grated parmesan cheese

Directions:

1. Preheat oven to 425°F (220°C). Line a rimmed 13 x 18 -inch (33 x 48 cm) baking sheet with aluminum foil or parchment paper.

2. Place tomatoes, chickpeas, garlic, canola oil, balsamic vinegar, and black pepper in a large bowl. Gently toss.

3. Place tomato mixture on prepared pan and roast for 15 minutes or until softened.

4. Meanwhile, in a large pot of boiling water cook pasta according to package directions. Pasta should be tender but

firm. Drain (do not rinse), reserving 1/2 cup (125 mL) of pasta water.

5. Place pasta in a large bowl, adding in roasted tomato mixture (be sure to get all the pan juices), reserved pasta water, and fresh basil. Gently toss.

6. Divide pasta into bowls and garnish with fresh basil leaves and cheese, if using.

Turkey Chili

Ingredients

1 pkg (500 g) lean ground turkey

10 mL (2 tsp) canola oil

1 onion, finely chopped

1 green pepper, chopped

4 cloves garlic, minced

15 mL (1 tbsp) chili powder

10 mL (2 tsp) dried oregano

5 mL (1 tsp) ground cumin

1 jalapeño pepper, seeded and minced

1 can (796 mL/28 oz) diced tomatoes

1 can (540 mL/19 oz) red kidney beans, drained and rinsed

125 mL (1/2 cup) sodium reduced vegetable broth or water

60 mL (1/4 cup) tomato paste

2 bay leaves

Directions:

1. In a large saucepan, brown turkey, breaking up with spoon. Drain using a colander and set aside. Return the empty pot to medium heat. Add oil and cook onion, green pepper, garlic, chili powder, oregano and cumin for about 3 minutes or until softened.

2. Stir in turkey and jalapeño pepper and cook, stirring for 1 minute.

3. Add tomatoes, beans, broth, tomato paste and bay leaves. Bring to a boil; reduce heat, cover slightly and simmer, stirring occasionally for about 20 minutes or until thickened. Remove bay leaves before serving

Vegan Chili

Ingredients

1 large onion, diced

3-4 cloves minced garlic

1 large green bell pepper, diced

1 large red bell pepper, diced

8oz your choice of meat substitutes

1 splash vegetable broth (for sautéing)

½ cup bulgur, uncooked

8oz can tomato sauce

15oz can fire-roasted diced tomatoes

1-2 Tbs masa harina (optional as a thickener)

2 Tbs pickled jalapeños (optional)

½ tsp garlic powder

2 cups low-sodium vegetable broth

1 cup refried beans

¼ cup McCormick's chili powder

2 tsp ground cumin

1 tsp paprika

1 tsp oregano

15oz can pinto beans (drained & rinsed))

15oz can kidney beans (not drained)

½ tsp black pepper

Instructions

1. Chop onions and peppers into a large soup pot or dutch oven

2. Saute in a little veggie broth until translucent and softened.

3. Add minced garlic and saute for an additional 30 seconds until fragrant

4. Add any kind of meat substitute (if using) or dry, uncooked bulgur and continue to stir for a few minutes until heated through

5. Add tomatoes, tomato sauce, and remaining broth

6. Add in spices and stir until mixed well

7. Add all the beans and jalapeños and stir

8. Sprinkle up to 1-2 Tbs of the Masa on top if you think it needs thickening. The masa adds a slight 'corn tortilla' or 'tamale' flavor to the chili.

9. Give the chili one more good stir and bring it to a slow boil.

10. Reduce heat, cover, and simmer for 15 to 30 minutes.

Sloppy Soy Curls

Ingredients

Soy Curls Marinade

3 cups Butler Soy Curls (dry)

2 cups Hot Water

2 Tbs Soy Sauce (low sodium)

½ tsp Garlic Powder ((optional)

½ tsp Onion Powder ((optional))

½ tsp Mrs Dash Seasoning ((optional))

Sloppy Joe Mix

8 oz Tomato Sauce

1 tsp Jalapeno (minced)

2 tsp Garlic (minced)

½ Onion (white)

1 Bell Pepper (red or green)

¼ cup Vegetable Broth (low sodium)

½ bottle Stubb's Original BBQ Sauce ((18 oz bottle)

1 tsp Red Wine Vinegar

Instructions

1. Add dry Soy Curls, hot water, and soy sauce to a large bowl and set aside. Stir occasionally.

2. Chop onion and bell pepper and saute in the vegetable broth until softened

3. Add garlic and jalapeño and cook for 1 minute

4. Drain soy curls, squeezing out any excess water, and chop finely. Add to pan with veggies and stir.

5. Add Tomato Sauce, BBQ Sauce, and Vinegar and stir.

6. Simmer over med heat until reduced to desired consistency.

Vegan Marinara Sauce

Ingredients

⅓ cup Leeks or Onions ((diced)

⅓ cup Red Bell Pepper ((diced)

⅓ cup White Mushrooms ((sliced)

2 cloves Garlic ((minced)

1 can Diced Tomatoes - No Salt Added ((15oz)

1 can Fire Roasted Chopped Tomatoes ((15oz))

1 can Tomato Paste ((6oz)

½ cup Red Wine

1 tsp Brown Sugar (or sweetener of choice) ((optional)

1 tsp Oregano

1 tsp Basil

1 tsp Parsley

¼ tsp Red Wine Vinegar

¼ tsp ground pepper

Salt to taste

Instructions

1. Finely dice the onion and bell pepper to a uniform size.

2. Sauté all the veggies together in a saucepan, just until they soften. Use a tablespoon or two of veg broth or water to prevent sticking if needed.

3. Add the sliced mushrooms and continue cooking until they have reduced in size and released their liquid.

4. Stir in the minced garlic and continue simmering for 1 minute or until fragrant.

5. Add the wine and stir to combine. Cook for 1-2 minutes. The wine adds a very elegant flavor to the sauce, but can be replaced with veg broth if necessary.

6. Add the tomatoes and tomato paste and mix thoroughly.

7. Add the remaining seasonings and simmer uncovered on low heat for about 30 minutes. The brown sugar is optional but helps reduce the overall acidity.

8. If the sauce is too chunky for your liking – you can use an immersion blender or....blend a cup or two, to get the consistency you like.

CHICKEN DIVAN

INGREDIENTS

5 cups broccoli florets

1 lb chicken breast, cubed

1/2 tsp sea salt

1/4 tsp black pepper

1 tbsp arrowroot starch

2 tbsp avocado oil

For the sauce

2 tbsp avocado oil

3 cloves garlic, minced

1 1/4 cup chicken broth

1 tbsp apple cider vinegar

1/3 cup coconut cream

1/3 tsp sea salt

1 tbsp + 2 tsp arrowroot starch

For topping

1 1/2 cup plantain chips (finely crushed, manually or with a food processor)

2 tbsp nutritional yeast

1 tbsp parsley, chopped

INSTRUCTIONS

1. Using a large deep pot, place the broccoli in a large pot with enough water to cover. Bring to a low boil and simmer for 5 minutes or until lightly fork tender. Strain and set aside in a large 9×13" casserole dish.

2. Season the chicken with salt and pepper and coat with arrowroot starch. Using a large pan, heat the avocado oil over medium heat. Cook the chicken in the pan for 4-5 minutes or until the internal temperature reads 165 F. Set the chicken aside.

3. Clean out the same pot used for the broccoli and heat the avocado oil over medium heat. Saute the garlic until fragrant.

4. Pour in the chicken broth (reserve 1/4 cup on the side), apple cider vinegar, coconut cream, and salt. Stir and bring to a low simmer.

5. Using a small bowl, whisk together the 1/4 cup of broth and the arrowroot starch. Pour into the broth mixture and stir well. Allow to simmer and thicken for 2-3 minutes. Set aside and allow to cool slightly.

6. Preheat the oven to 400 F. Add the chicken to the casserole dish with the broccoli and stir to evenly disperse.

7. Pour the sauce over the chicken and broccoli and top with the finely crushed plantain chips and nutritional yeast.

8. Bake in the preheated oven for 15-18 minutes or until the top is crispy.

9. Top with fresh parsley and serve with cauliflower rice if desired

Veggie Papas with Red Chile Sauce

Ingredients

1 bag Simply Potatoes (1 lb 4 oz) ((or 4 cups shredded))

1 cup Mushrooms (diced small)

¼ tsp Black Pepper

½ tsp Onion Powder

½ tsp Garlic Powder

2 cups New Mexican Red Chile Sauce

½ cup Tomatoes (diced small)

½ cup Green Bell Pepper (diced small)

½ cup Yellow Onion (diced small)

Instructions

1. Prepare Red Chile Sauce

2. Preheat oven to 450 degrees F.

3. If shredding potatoes manually, be sure and squeeze any excess moisture out of them before continuing. Otherwise, place potatoes into a large bowl.

4. Add veggies and spices and mix thoroughly.

5. Turn potatoes out onto a parchment-lined baking sheet and spread evenly. Press down a little to compress (helps them stick together).

6. Bake for 30 minutes or until the edges are nice and crispy.

7. Serve with warm Red Chile Sauce over the top.

Stroke of Midnight

INGREDIENTS

1 green cardamom pod

9 oz. gin

9 oz. Lillet Blanc

4½ oz. filtered water

1 oz. unaged pear brandy (such as Clear Creek)

Lemon twists (for serving)

INSTRUCTIONS

In a quart-size jar, muddle 1 green cardamom pod to break it up. Add 9 oz. gin, 9 oz. Lillet Blanc, 4½ oz. filtered water, and 1 oz. unaged pear brandy (such as Clear Creek). Refrigerate for 24 hours.

Strain off cardamom pod using a fine-mesh strainer. Pour mixture back into jar and return to refrigerator until 1 hour before serving.

One hour before serving, move jar to freezer to chill. When ready to serve, pour into Nick and Nora or martini glasses and garnish with lemon twists.

Heart-Healthy Chopped Potato Breakfast Salad

INGREDIENTS

Salad Ingredients

3 large potatoes, scrubbed and cut into 3/4-inch cubes; approx. 3 cups

Cooking spray

6 egg whites

1 cup chopped red pepper

1 cup canned chickpeas (garbanzo beans) (rinsed, drained)

Dressing Ingredients

1 cup fresh parsley, chopped (packed into cup measure)

2 tablespoons olive oil, extra virgin

2 tablespoons fresh lemon juice

1 tablespoon real maple syrup

INSTRUCTIONS

1. Place potato cubes in a large saucepan; add water to cover and bring to boil over medium-high heat. Boil potatoes for 5 minutes, or until tender (easily pierced with a knife). Drain and place in a serving bowl.

2. Lightly spray a nonstick skillet with cooking spray. Cook the egg whites over medium heat, without stirring, until cooked through but not overcooked. Flip skillet over onto a clean cutting board, releasing egg whites. Chop egg whites and add to serving bowl.

3. Add red pepper and chickpeas to the bowl, stirring all ingredients to combine; set aside. Prepare dressing: Puree all ingredients in a blender. Add to salad and toss gently to combine.

Sweet Potato Avocado Toasts with Walnuts

INGREDIENTS

2 sweet potatoes

2 avocados (thinly sliced)

1/2 cup walnuts (diced)

1½ tsp red pepper flakes, plus more if desired

4 teaspoons extra virgin olive oil

3/4 teaspoon flaky salt

INSTRUCTIONS

1. Slice a small plank off one side of each sweet potato lengthwise. This will act as a base, so you can cut the sweet potato into toast slices easily. Prop the sweet potato on the flat side you created and slice each potato into planks about ¼ inch thick.

2. For toaster preparation, pop the sweet potato planks in the toaster and toast until tender. This may take a few times, depending on your toaster.

3. For oven preparation, preheat your oven to 350° F. Lay the sweet potato planks on a baking sheet and spray with cooking spray. Roast for 6-7 minutes per side, until they are easily pierced with a fork.

4. When they're done toasting, lay the sweet potato toasts on plates and top with sliced avocado. Mash the avocado gently with a fork. Sprinkle with diced walnuts, red pepper flakes and drizzle with olive oil. Top with flaky salt.

Hearty and Heart-Healthy Potato Soup

INGREDIENTS

2 pounds potatoes, scrubbed and cut in 1/2-inch cubes (about 5 cups)

1 tablespoon olive oil

2 10-ounce packages frozen chopped onions

1/4 cup chopped, dried tomatoes

2 pints plus 1 14-ounce can (46 ounces total) low-sodium chicken broth

2 cups shredded, cooked turkey

3 cups packaged, chopped, frozen mixed vegetables, thawed

freshly-ground black pepper

INSTRUCTIONS

1. In heavy soup pot, heat oil on high and stir in onions. Cook, stirring occasionally for about 20 minutes or until well browned.

2. Add potatoes, dried tomatoes and broth.

3. Bring to boil and cook covered for 10 minutes or until tender.

4. Add turkey and vegetables, return to boil and cook 6 - 8 minutes.

5. Top with freshly ground pepper.

Mustard - Homemade Condiments

INGREDIENTS

4 Tbsp. ground mustard

1 tsp. sugar

1/4 tsp. salt

1/4 cup white vinegar

1/8 tsp. paprika

1/8 tsp. turmeric

1 tsp. cornstarch

INSTRUCTIONS

1. In a jar that holds 1 cup mix the ground mustard, sugar, salt, vinegar, paprika and turmeric. Cover and microwave for 30-40 seconds.

2. Add cornstarch to heated mustard mixture ½ teaspoon at a time and mix well.

3. Store in the refrigerator in a covered jar.

Shrimp Ceviche

INGREDIENTS

1 garlic clove

1 jalapeño pepper

1/2 cup lime juice (fresh)

2 Roma tomato

1 small red onion

1 avocado

1/2 bunch fresh cilantro

1 pound shrimp (peeled, steamed)

1 mango (peeled)

black pepper (to taste)

INSTRUCTIONS

1. Using the food processor, chop the garlic clove, jalapeño, Roma tomatoes, and red onion. You can add the lime juice if you need a little liquid to allow the processor to do its job. Place in a large mixing bowl.

2. With a knife chop the cilantro, shrimp, mango, and avocado and add it to the mixing bowl. (Do not put these items in food processor, please chop by hand)

3. Mix all the ingredients together (including any of the lime juice you didn't already add). Add the black pepper to taste.

Fish Fillets with Fresh Tomatoes

INGREDIENTS

2 Tbsp. olive oil (extra virgin preferred)

1 large rib of celery, chopped

1/3 cup chopped onion

3 large garlic cloves, crushed or minced

10-12 oz. Italian plum (Roma) tomatoes (chopped)

1 small carrot (thinly sliced)

1 small dried bay leaf

1/4 tsp. pepper

1/8 tsp. (heaping) ground cinnamon

1/8 tsp. salt

4 thin, mild fish fillets, such as sole, cod or tilapia (about 4 ounces each), rinsed, patted dry

1 1/2-2 Tbsp. fresh lemon juice

chopped parsley (optional)

INSTRUCTIONS

1. In a large skillet, heat the oil over medium heat, swirling to coat the bottom. Cook the celery, onion, and garlic for about 2 minutes, stirring constantly, adjusting the heat if necessary so the mixture doesn't brown. Stir in the tomatoes, carrot, bay leaf, pepper, cinnamon, and salt. Cook for 5 minutes.

2. Make 4 depressions in the tomato mixture. Place the fish in the depressions. Spoon the tomato mixture over the fish to cover. Cook for 3 to 5 minutes, or until the fish is almost done (there should be just a little resistance when you try to flake the fish with a fork). Remove from the heat.

3. Drizzle the fish with the lemon juice. Let stand, covered, for about 5 minutes so the fish finishes cooking and the flavors blend. Discard the bay leaf. Garnish with the parsley.

Cozy Beef Stew

INGREDIENTS

4 pounds boneless sirloin steak, all visible fat discarded, cut into 1-inch cubes

4 cups baby red potatoes, halved

4 cups baby carrots

2 medium onions, chopped

2 cups chopped celery

1 15-ounce can no-salt-added tomato sauce

10 ounces dried lima beans, sorted for stones and shriveled beans, rinsed, and drained

OR

10 ounces dried black-eyed peas, sorted for stones and shriveled peas, rinsed, and drained

2 tablespoons brown sugar

1 tablespoon plus 1 teaspoon quick-cooking tapioca

2 teaspoons pepper

1 teaspoon celery salt

1 teaspoon dried parsley, crumbled

1 teaspoon dried thyme, crumbled

1 cup water

INSTRUCTIONS

1. If frozen, thaw the bags in the refrigerator overnight. Pour the contents into a slow cooker. Stir in the water. Cook, covered, on low for 4 to 6 hours, or until the vegetables are tender.

Directions for Freezing

1. In a large bowl, stir together all the ingredients except the water. Transfer the mixture equally between two 1-gallon resealable plastic freezer bags. Lay the bags flat in the freezer.

ANIMAL COCKTAIL

Ingredients

FOR THE COCKTAIL

1 oz spiced rum

0.5 oz Caribbean Citrus Syrup

1/2 fresh lemon, juiced (approx 0.5 oz)

2 drops orange blossom water

sparkling wine to taste

FOR THE SYRUP

1/2 cup dark brown sugar

1/2 cup water

3-4 drops maple extract

1 dash fresh nutmeg

1/2 teaspoon

INSTRUCTIONS

To make syrup:

Combine all ingredients in a small saucepan. Bring to a boil, simmer for 5 minutes, strain, and cool.

To make the cocktail:

Pour ingredients into a cocktail shaker with ice. Shake cocktail and strain into a champagne flute without ice. Garnish with a slice of dehydrated blood orange.

Lemon Pepper Fish

INGREDIENTS

1lb fresh pickerel, perch, haddock, or walleye

1 ½ tsp lemon zest

½ tsp pepper

½ tsp salt, divided

1 carrot, thinly sliced

1 small zucchini, thinly sliced

2 tbsp chopped sun-dried tomatoes in oil

2 tbsp canola oil

2 tbsp white wine

1 tbsp lemon juice

1 garlic clove, rasped

Pinch each dried oregano and basil leaves

INSTRUCTIONS

1.   Place fish fillets in parchment paper lined 13 x 9 inch baking pan. Sprinkle with lemon, pepper, and ¼ tsp of the salt. Sprinkle with carrot, zucchini and tomatoes.

2.   In a small bowl, whisk together oil, wine, lemon juice, garlic, oregano, basil, and remaining salt. Drizzle over top of vegetables.

3.   Roast in 400 degrees Fahrenheit oven for about 20 minutes or until fish flakes when tested and ve:getables are lightly golden.

Apple Pie Oat Muffins

INGREDIENTS

3 cups large flake oats

2 tbsp ground cinnamon

2 tsp baking powder

¼ tsp salt

1 ½ cups milk

2 eggs

½ cup unsweetened apple sauce

¼ cup canola oil

¾ cup diced apple

¼ cup raisins

DIRECTIONS

1.   In a large bowl, combine oats, cinnamon, baking powder and salt.

2.   In another bowl, whisk together milk, eggs, apple sauce and oil. Pour over oat mixture and stir to combine. Stir in apple and raisins.

3.   Divide mixture among 12 lightly sprayed muffin tins. Bake in preheated 350 degrees Fahrenheit oven for about 30 minutes or until tester inserted in centre comes out clean.

4.   Serve warm as is or with a drizzle of maple syrup.

Chicken Tzatziki Pita

INGREDIENTS

Chopped cooked chicken 2 cups (500 mL)

Spinach ½ cup, lightly packed

Green onions, chopped 2

Small red, green, orange or yellow bell pepper, chopped 1

Shredded light cheddar cheese ½ cup (125 mL)

Tzatziki ¼ cup (60 mL)

Hot pepper sauce (optional) ¼ tsp (1 mL)

Large whole wheat flour tortillas x 4

DIRECTIONS

1. In a bowl, combine chicken, spinach, onions, pepper, cheese, tzatziki and hot pepper sauce, if using.

2. Stuff pitas with chicken mixture.

Chicken Fried Rice

INGREDIENTS

1/2 cup instant brown rice

2 tsp sesame oil

1 large red onion (diced)

2 large carrots (peeled and diced)

6 ounces boneless skinless chicken thighs (cubed)

1 tsp ground ginger

2/3 cup frozen peas (thawed)

fresh ground black pepper (to taste)

3 tsp low sodium soy or gluten-free tamari sauce

1 large egg (beaten)

DIRECTIONS

1. Cook the instant brown rice to the directions on the package.

2. When the rice is ready, set it aside. Place the sesame oil in a wok or large skillet over high heat. When the oil is very hot and nearly smoking, add the onions and carrots. Cook for about 3 to 4 minutes until the onions begin to soften.

3. Add the chicken thighs and ginger. Cook for about ten minutes, stirring frequently. Add the peas, pepper and soy or tamari sauce.

4. Add the cooked rice and toss until the rice, veggies and chicken are well blended.

5. Add the beaten egg and toss until the egg is cooked through. Serve.

Caprese Frittatas

INGREDIENTS

6 eggs

85 mL (⅓ cup) skim milk or unsweetened plant-based beverages

2 mL (½ tsp) salt

2 mL (½ tsp) pepper

2 tomatoes, chopped finely

5 mL (1 tsp) dried basil

125 mL (½ cup) grated low fat mozzarella cheese

½ cup sautéed spinach (optional)

DIRECTIONS

1. Preheat the oven to 400° F. Lightly spray or paper-line 6 muffin tins.

2. In a large bowl, whisk together eggs, milk, salt and pepper. Add tomatoes and basil and whisk well.

3. Using a 125 mL (½ cup) measuring cup, scoop batter into muffin tins until divided evenly. Add 15 mL (1 tbsp) of grated cheese on top of each frittata.

4. Cook frittatas in the oven for about 15 minutes. Use a digital food thermometer to check that the eggs have reached an internal temperature of 74° C (165° F).

5. Let cool for 3 – 5 minutes before removing from muffin tins.

Chicken Fajitas

INGREDIENTS

400 grams boneless, skinless, chicken breasts

10 mL (2 tsp) chili powder

2 mL (1/2 tsp) ground cumin

2 mL (1/2 tsp) fresh ground pepper

10 mL (2 tsp) canola oil, divided

1 onion, thinly sliced

2 red, orange or yellow bell peppers, thinly sliced

75 mL (1/3 cup) chopped fresh cilantro

6 small whole grain or corn tortillas or pitas

Lime Crema:

60 mL (1/4 cup) light sour cream or plain Greek yogurt.

2 mL (1/2 tsp) grated lime rind

30 mL (2 tbsp) lime juice

DIRECTIONS

1. Using a large knife, thinly slice chicken crosswise into thin strips. Toss with chili powder, cumin and pepper.

2. In a nonstick skillet, heat half of the oil over medium high heat and brown chicken. Remove to plate. Add remaining oil in same skillet and sauté onion, bell peppers and cilantro for 4 minutes or until tender crisp. Return chicken to skillet and heat through.

3. For the lime crema, in a small bowl, stir together sour cream, lime rind and lime juice.

4. Divide chicken-veggie mixture among tortillas and top with lime sour crema.

Creamy Lemon Dill White Bean Dip

INGREDIENTS

1 15 ounce can white beans, drained and rinsed

1 cup fresh dill (loosely packed)

1 lemon, juiced (or more to taste)

¼ cup avocado oil

1 clove garlic (optional)

¾ teaspoon of fine sea salt

¼ teaspoon ground black pepper

lemon zest for garnish

INSTRUCTIONS

1. Place all ingredients in a mini food processor (or regular food processor) and begin to process until smooth and creamy.

2. Taste and adjust seasonings to your liking (you might want to add more salt, pepper, garlic, lemon or dill). If you want the dip to be thinner, add one tablespoon of warm water.

3. Transfer dip to a bowl and garnish with lemon zest and a sprig of fresh dill. Serve with fresh veggies (radishes, carrots, celery, bell peppers or cucumbers), chips, warm gluten-free pita bread or crackers.

SPINACH ARTICHOKE CHICKEN SKILLET

Ingredients

For the chicken breast:

4 small-medium boneless skinless chicken breast or 2 large halved

1 tablespoon basil

1 tablespoon garlic powder

1 teaspoon sea salt

1/2 teaspoon black pepper

1 tablespoon ghee (or olive oil)

For the creamy sauce:

1 tablespoon ghee (or olive oil)

3 cloves garlic, minced

1 yellow onion, finely chopped

1/4 cup chicken broth

1 13.5–ounce can unsweetened full-fat coconut milk, (I recommend Thai Kitchen Coconut Milk)

1/2 lemon, juiced

1 tablespoon arrowroot starch

1/2 teaspoon salt

1/4 teaspoon black pepper

1 14–ounce can quartered artichoke hearts, drained and chopped

2 cups packed spinach

red pepper flakes, garnish

Instructions

1. Season the chicken breast on both sides with basil, garlic powder, salt and black pepper. Heat oil over medium heat in skillet. Sauté chicken breast on each side for 6-8 minutes. Transfer cooked chicken breast to a plate.

2. In the same skillet (just remove the brown bits left if they're too dark), over medium heat, melt ghee. Add garlic and onions, and sauté over medium heat for 1-2 minutes.

3. Add the chicken broth, coconut milk, lemon juice, arrowroot, salt, and pepper to the skillet. Whisk together. Simmer for 2-3 minutes or until sauce thickens. Reduce heat to low. Stir in artichoke hearts and spinach. Return the chicken to the skillet, and spoon the sauce over the chicken. Garnish with red pepper flakes. Serve hot.

CREAMY TURKEY MUSHROOM SOUP

INGREDIENTS

2 tablespoons oil

10 ounces mushrooms, sliced

1 medium onion, chopped

4 cloves garlic, minced

2 medium carrots, chopped

2 stalks celery, chopped

1 medium potato, peeled and cut in half

1 teaspoon dried thyme

6 cups homemade turkey stock, can sub chicken

2 cups shredded turkey meat, can sub chicken

¼ cup cashews, see notes

 Sea salt and pepper, to taste

INSRUCTIONS

Note: this recipe uses the leftover meat from your turkey dinner and stock made from the bones. You need to make the stock first – it's easy!

Heat the oil in a large pot over medium-high heat. Add the mushrooms and cook until they are soft and starting to brown, about 10 minutes. Add the onion and cook until it softens, about 3-4 minutes. Add the garlic and cook for 1 minute more.

2 tablespoons oil,10 ounces mushrooms,1 medium onion,4 cloves garlic

Add the carrots, celery, potato, thyme, turkey stock, and meat to the pot and bring to a boil. Reduce to heat to medium and simmer the soup for 20 minutes, or until the potato is soft.

2 medium carrots,2 stalks celery,1 medium potato,1 teaspoon dried thyme,6 cups homemade turkey stock,2 cups shredded turkey meat

Remove the two potato halves from the soup and put them in your blender. Add the cashews and enough of the soup liquid so they will blend. Don't worry if you get a few small pieces of the other veggies into your blender. Blend on high until smooth then return the 'cream' to the pot. Season to taste with sea salt and pepper.

¼ cup cashews

Gluten Free Biscuits

Ingredients

2 cups All-Purpose Gluten Free Flour

1 teaspoon Xanthan Gum

1 teaspoon Fine Sea Salt

2 1/2 teaspoons Baking Powder

6 tablespoons Butter, Cubed and cold

3/4 cup Milk

Instructions

1. Preheat the oven to 425°F.

2. In a large bowl, whisk together the flour, xanthan gum, salt and baking powder. Use a pastry cutter to cut the butter into the flour mixture until it resembles coarse cornmeal.

3. Stir in the milk until incorporated. You may need an additional 1-2 tablespoons of milk to insure all the flour is moistened. Form the dough into a ball and knead about 10 times in the bowl.

4. Roll the dough out on a floured board to desired thickness (biscuits will not rise much while baking). I roll the dough to about 1 ½ - 2 inches thick. Use a 2 inch biscuit cutter to cut the biscuits. Gently re-roll dough as needed.

5. Place biscuits on an ungreased baking sheet and refrigerate for 30 minutes (uncovered) before baking. You can also make the dough a few hours ahead of time and leave refrigerated until ready to bake.

6. After 30 minutes chilling, bake 12-15 minutes or until done (cooking time will depend on thickness of the biscuit). Serve warm.

7. Store leftovers in an air-tight container or bag overnight or freeze.

Smoky Maple Tofu Bacon

Ingredients

1 block Extra Firm Tofu (14oz)

¼ cup Soy Sauce (low sodium)

2 Tbs Maple Syrup

1 Tbs Nutritional Yeast

2 tsp Liquid Smoke

1 tsp Onion Powder

½ tsp Garlic Powder

Instructions

1. Drain tofu , wrap the block in paper towels, and press under something heavy to remove as much moisture as possible. Let press for 15 minutes.

2. Carefully slice tofu lengthwise into ⅛" slices. I have used a cheese slicer and a mandolin with good success. Just be careful.

3. Whisk all remaining ingredients together in a small bowl to make the marinade.

4. Lay the slices of tofu flat in large pan or dish and cover with marinade. Let the tofu marinate for at least 15 minutes, preferably 30 min to 1 hr.

5. To broil: Place the tofu slices on a foil lined baking sheet and place under your broiler. Turn occasionally to brown both sides.

Note: Do not use parchment paper.

6. To pan fry: Place the slices in a non-stick skillet and cook on med-high heat until browned, flipping occasionally. If the tofu appears to be sticking, pour a little water in the pan to loosen.

Creamy Vegan Mac and Cheese

Ingredients

16 oz Yukon Gold Potatoes (about 3 medium)

1-2 Carrots

½ cup Water

¼ cup + 2 Tbs Nutritional yeast

2 Tbs Lemon Juice

1 tsp Apple Cider Vinegar

1 tsp Salt

½ tsp Onion Powder

½ tsp Garlic Powder

½ tsp Brown or Yellow Mustard

¼ tsp Turmeric

2 cups Elbow Macaroni

1 bag Frozen Broccoli (a 12oz bag)

Instructions

1. Wash and scrub both potatoes and carrots, peel if desired.

2. Chop into uniform pieces and boil for 10 minutes.

INSTANT POT: Or - simply add them to your Instant Pot with 1 cup of water. Set to MANUAL and cook for 7 minutes. Allow to naturally release for 10 minutes before opening lid.

3. Remove from heat and let rest for 5 minutes

4. With a slotted spoon, transfer veggies to a blender

5. Add ½ cup of the hot potato water (more if needed to blend smoothly)

6. Pulse to mix

7. Add in remaining ingredients and blend until smooth

8. Boil pasta until al dente

9. Add in frozen vegetables to last 5 min of boiling

10. Drain pasta, return to pan, and stir in however much cheese sauce you like until creamy and evenly coated

Peanut Noodles

Ingredients

¼ cup low-sodium soy sauce

¼ cup water

1-2 tablespoons minced garlic

1 tablespoon rice vinegar

1 tablespoon maple syrup

2-3 tablespoons peanut butter or PB2

¼ tsp ground ginger

7 oz rice noodles (½ package Thai kitchen brand rice noodles)

11 oz package frozen vegetables (broccoli & cauliflower)

Optional Additions:

1 tablespoon hoisin sauce

½ to 1 tsp sriracha or other hot sauce

8 oz mushrooms

Optional Garnishes:

chopped green onions

sesame seeds

sriracha

Instructions

1. In a small saucepan, combine all the sauce ingredients.

2. Heat over low heat until bubbly.

3. Bring about ½ a pasta pot of water to a boil.

4. Add the noodles and cook per package instructions

5. Microwave frozen veggies per package instructions (or add frozen veggies to the boiling pasta water if you do not want to microwave)

6. Drain completely, stir in sauce, and serve.

Conclusions

A stroke can be a life-changing event, but with proper nutrition and lifestyle changes, it is possible to recover and regain health and wellness. The Stroke Recovery Cookbook offers a range of delicious and nutritious recipes to help individuals recovering from stroke improve their overall health and wellbeing.

By focusing on easy and nutritious breakfasts, nourishing soups and stews, power-packed salads, flavorful and lean proteins, and practical meal planning and prep, this cookbook provides a comprehensive approach to stroke recovery nutrition. With recipes that are both delicious and healthy, individuals can enjoy their meals while also supporting their recovery.

Furthermore, the practical tips and advice provided throughout the cookbook make it easy to simplify the recovery diet and make meal planning and prep a breeze. By following the guidelines in this cookbook, individuals can ensure they are getting the nutrients they need to heal and recover.

Overall, The Stroke Recovery Cookbook is an excellent resource for anyone recovering from stroke and looking to improve their health and wellbeing through nutritious and delicious meals. With a focus on practicality, taste, and health, this cookbook offers a comprehensive approach to stroke recovery nutrition that is sure to support individuals in their journey towards optimal health and wellness.